HEALTHCARE CAREER AS AN

ALLERGIST

ALLERGY, ASTHMA PECIALIST

DOCTORS, NURSES, TECHNICIANS

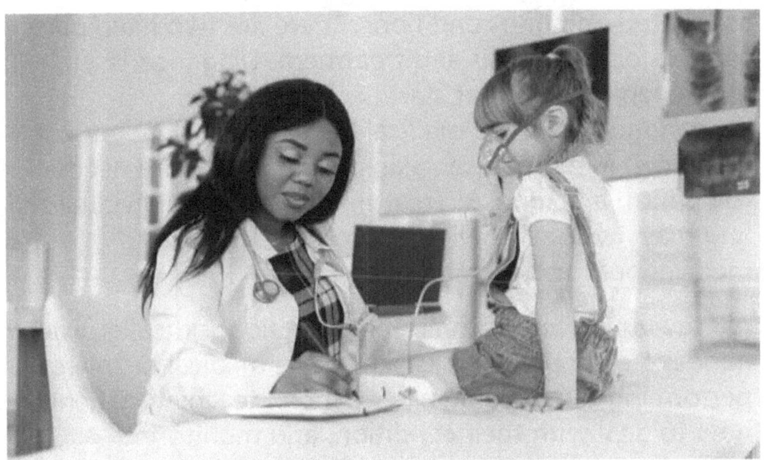

IT IS ESTIMATED THAT 50 MILLION AMERICANS are affected by allergies and/or asthma. Sneezing, coughing, headaches, stomach pains, and hives are among the most common symptoms. They are the result of the body's immune response to foreign substances, known as allergens or triggers. We are all familiar with the term "hay fever," which is an allergic reaction to pollen. Anything can trigger an allergic response, including certain foods, animals, medicines, or even sunshine and water.

Most allergies are minor and can be alleviated with a combination of avoidance and over-the-counter medications. Others are more serious. They may interfere with daily activities and require medical attention. Some are even life threatening. Allergy specialists can help people regain their ability to enjoy life without worry of when the next allergy attack will hit.

Allergy specialists, including allergists, allergy nurses, and allergy technicians, have specific training in the field of allergies. Allergists are board-certified physicians who are capable of managing a full range of allergies and associated immune conditions. There are two main parts to their job: diagnosis and treatment. Diagnosis is a multi-step process that starts with a physical examination, detailed medical history, and a patient interview. In many cases, skin or blood tests are needed to confirm a diagnosis. Treatment plans are individualized and may involve lifestyle changes, prescription medications, and/or immunotherapy.

Allergy nurses and technicians work alongside allergists, handling a variety of tasks like taking medical histories, performing tests, giving allergy shots, teaching patients how to deal with their condition, and monitoring patients' conditions over time. They can do just about anything the allergist does, except determine a diagnosis and develop a treatment plan. Working together, the team can improve a patient's overall quality of life.

There is a growing need for allergy specialists that shows no signs of slowing down. The occurrence of allergic diseases has risen sharply over the past 50 years. Many allergy disorders, especially the newest ones, need the expertise of an allergy specialist. Yet, there are not enough of these specialized professionals to meet the demand. There is a growing shortage that is fueling a faster-than-average employment growth.

The outlook is very good for those entering the field. That means there will be plenty of job opportunities just about anywhere in the country. Although there are some hospitals with allergy specialists on staff, most jobs are in private practices providing outpatient services. Emergencies are virtually unheard of, and overtime is rare. A standard 9 to 5 schedule is the norm.

Like most doctors, allergists are paid well. In fact, they are currently experiencing the second fastest salary growth of all doctors. The average salary is $250,000 a year and there is potential to earn much more.

Also, like most doctors, it takes years of rigorous education and training to become an allergist. The undergraduate work, medical school, residency, and fellowship required to become a board-certified allergist adds up to 13 years.

Training is also required for allergy nurses and technicians, but not nearly as much. Allergy nurses are registered nurses (RNs) with specific knowledge of allergy treatment and management. They can get started with as little as two to three years of full-time training. Although not required, allergy RNs can also obtain professional certification. With certification and experience, allergy nurses can earn up to $95,000 per year.

Allergy technicians often perform the same tasks as allergy nurses, but they can get started with even less time spent in school. Few states have any educational requirements for allergy technicians, but most employers do want to see at least a one-year certificate or two-year associate degree in medical technology or a related field.

Like allergy nurses, technicians can add to their qualifications by obtaining certification that will impress prospective employers. Considering the minimal requirements, allergy technicians are paid well. The national average stands at $45,000.

If you can handle the educational requirements and have a desire to help as many people as possible, this could be a good career choice. It comes loaded with benefits, marked by a high level of job and personal satisfaction and the opportunity to make an enormous difference in people's lives. Since patients are everywhere, you do not need to relocate to find a job. Once school is in the past, you can look forward to the kind of work/life balance most medical professionals envy.

WHAT YOU CAN DO NOW

MEMBERS OF THE ALLERGY HEALTHCARE TEAM need to be well-educated. It takes 13 years of rigorous training to head up the team as a board certified allergist. Nurses and technicians do not need to spend that much time in school, but they do need more than a high school diploma. Check with your guidance counselor to make sure you have all the necessary courses to meet college admissions requirements.

Your high school curriculum should include a full four years each of English, mathematics, and sciences (including biology and chemistry). Make your high school record stand out by taking challenging courses in mathematics. Consider taking advanced placement (AP) courses in biology and chemistry. If you do well, you may receive college credit for those classes, but at least it will look good on your admission application.

Good communications are important in this field. Consider taking extra classes, such as debate and English composition, which will help boost your speaking and writing skills. Classes in computer science are a plus.

Many top universities conduct summer study programs for high school students who are preparing for careers in medicine. These are usually tuition-free, residential programs that last about a month. They are designed to improve participants' academic study skills in preparation for the intense postsecondary education that lies ahead.

There are also summer study programs specifically focused on the field of allergic and immunologic diseases. For example, NIAID laboratories in Maryland and Montana offer two-month summer interns the chance to perform full-time biomedical research into these diseases. This is an exceptional opportunity to work with members of the National Institute of Health's research team.

Explore the career to make sure it is a good fit for you. Talk to allergy healthcare specialists in your community. You can find them by calling hospitals or searching sites like LinkedIn. Your guidance counselor may be helpful in making connections, too. Try to arrange at least one job shadow to see what working in the field is really like.

HISTORY OF THE PROFESSION

ALLERGIES ARE NOT NEW. IN FACT, they have probably plagued humans forever. Common allergic symptoms, such as runny noses, rashes, and especially respiratory distress, have been described in ancient documents of China and Egypt as far back as 2600 B.C. However, it would take 2,000 years before there was any understanding of them.

Hippocrates, the father of Western medicine, linked the symptoms of asthma to environmental triggers associated with specific trades. He did not define or name the disease. That would take another 600 years. Around 100 AD, an important Greek Physician and medical writer known as Aretaeus of Cappadocia, was the first to accurately describe asthma and how it develops. He also gave it a name. Asthma is derived from the Greek word aazein, which means "panting."

Around the same time, symptoms of other allergic diseases were being explored in ancient Rome. Pliny the Elder, a prolific author and philosopher, linked pollen and breathing problems. Unlike Hippocrates, he recommended a treatment which was a predecessor of epinephrine. Roman philosopher Lucretius also wrote in the first century AD, "What is food to one man is bitter poison to others." While this proved to be an important medical breakthrough, it would take many exhaustive studies over centuries to pin down the cause and effect of food allergies.

In the Middle Ages, physicians discovered that some flowers, such as roses, caused allergic reactions, such as excessive sneezing. Renaissance doctors sought methods of preventing allergies, which had the unexpected benefit of identifying various sources of allergies. Early in the 1600s, the term "summer asthma" was used to describe seasonal allergies. The term "hay fever" was not used until the late 1700s.

Modern understanding of allergies began to slowly take shape in the 19th century. Dr. John Bostock, an American physician, wrote the first detailed description of hay fever – the most common allergic issue to this day. Picking up the investigation in the 1860s, English doctor, Charles Harrison Blackley, was determined to identify the cause of his own bouts of hay fever. He rejected popular theories of the time, such as heat and ozone. After extensive experiments on himself, he was able to prove that the culprit was pollen. Unfortunately, he was unable to come up with an effective treatment, but he did develop the first skin test for allergies.

Meanwhile, British doctor Henry Hyde Salter wrote his historically acclaimed book, *On Asthma: Its Pathology and Treatment.* In addition to proposing remedies, the book included medical drawings of the lungs and detailed descriptions of what happens during asthma attacks.

Near the close of the 19th century, one of the co-founders of the John Hopkins Medical School named Sir William Osler, conducted the most significant research to date into the causes and treatment of asthma. He noted links between asthma and allergic conditions that affect the respiratory system. In terms of causes, Osler considered the possibility that asthma could be hereditary, and identified specific triggers like stress and diet.

Osler's most important research, however, proved that the airway blockage during an asthma attack was the result of smooth muscle spasms. This discovery led to pharmacies distributing bronchodilators that could calm airway spasms and increase airflow to the lungs during asthma attacks.

20th Century and the Modern Concept of Allergies

The word "allergy" was used for the first time in 1906 by Clemens von Pirquet. The Austrian pediatrician had noticed that second doses of horse serum or smallpox vaccines caused quick and severe reactions in some patients. He correctly concluded that this was the result of the immune system producing antibodies to fight off foreign substances contained within the serum.

Following up on this concept over the next few years, researchers discovered that the same hypersensitive reaction of the immune system was indeed an allergic reaction. Further studies involving immunotherapy found a link between the most extreme allergic reaction (anaphylaxis) and the body's production of the chemical histamine. This was a huge step forward. By 1914, allergy clinics were offering to help patients overcome allergies through gradual exposure to specific antigens.

In the late 1930s, the first antihistamines were developed. These medications helped lessen the body's reaction to allergens. Corticosteroids, which were discovered a decade later, were proven effective in treating both allergic reactions and asthma by reducing inflammation. Soon after, anti-allergy products, such as non-biological washing powder, began appearing on store shelves. Food labeling was initiated along with warnings about potential allergies.

Allergy research intensified in the 1960s. Previously, all forms of hypersensitivity were considered to be the same at their core. This was proven false, and as a result allergies were reclassified into different types. However, in 1967, researchers discovered that one particular antibody was responsible for most allergic reactions. The antibody labeled immunoglobulin E (IgE) was the specific antibody that produced the process of sensitization upon exposure to an antigen, whether it was peanuts, pollen, or any other allergy-inducing chemical.

In the 1960s through the 1980's, there was an over reliance on bronchodilators that had dire consequences. The medications, which were considered standard treatment, were only good for short-term soothing. By disregarding longer-term management, doctors failed to address the deeper immune problems behind asthma.

The result was an epidemic of asthma deaths. In an effort to reverse this surge of mortality among asthma sufferers, researchers got back to work looking for more effective treatments. Clinical trials produced corticosteroids that could provide effective daily management and control of asthma. Other developments included blood tests to detect IgE levels and the EpiPen to treat anaphylactic shock.

Today, asthma and allergies are the sixth leading cause of chronic illness. The healthcare costs are astronomical at more than $18 billion a year, so more research is needed. Despite progress in the treatment and management of allergy symptoms, a cure does not yet exist. There are effective tests for allergies and treatment options for minimizing the symptoms, and future treatments might involve altering genes and targeting immune cells with precision. For now, allergies and asthma are still mysterious, complex, and incurable conditions.

There are currently about 4,400 board certified allergists in the US. Most choose to work in clinical practice, which puts them in either private medical offices or hospitals. Those in private practice may be self-employed, running their own businesses. They may also be in partnerships with other doctors who practice different specialties.

In most cases, allergists who see patients in a hospital setting are actually solo practitioners who work with hospitals on a consulting basis. However, there are a variety of hospitals that have allergists on staff. Some are large general hospitals, both private and public. Others may be open to specific populations. For example, an allergist specializing in pediatric allergies and asthma would likely work at a children's hospital. There are also some allergists who work at teaching hospitals where they can combine patient care with occasional research projects and/or teaching.

Allergy specialists involved primarily in research do not typically work directly with patients. Their non-clinical work is conducted in laboratories. They may be employed by medical schools or government research facilities like the NIAID. Some are hired by private industry laboratories to work on the development of pharmaceuticals or medical equipment related to allergies and asthma.

Most allergy nurses and technicians work in clinical practice under the direction of a physician who is a board certified allergist. Most work in medical offices and some work in hospitals. It is rare to find them in laboratories.

Working Conditions

Once all training, including internships and residencies, are over, allergists enjoy a more flexible work schedule than some other kinds of doctors. They usually work full time on weekdays without much deviation in schedules since emergencies are extremely rare.

THE WORK YOU WILL DO

ALLERGY SPECIALISTS ARE TRAINED TO diagnose, manage, and treat a full range of allergies and associated immune conditions. Many allergies are mild and can be controlled with over-the-counter medications. Others can interfere with daily activities and decrease the quality of life. Some allergies can even be life threatening.

Allergies occur when an individual's immune system overreacts to a foreign substance, such as certain foods, pollen, pet dander, bee venom, dust mites, or chemicals. The substance that causes the allergic reaction is known as an allergen. When the allergen comes in contact with the body, the immune system produces antibodies that travel to cells that will release certain chemicals, such as histamines, that will cause an allergic reaction. Allergic symptoms usually cause inflammation at the site of the allergen contact. This could be the skin, stomach lining, eyes, ears, or any part of the respiratory system.

Most allergy specialists are generalists, accepting patients of all ages and conditions. The conditions they see the most often include:

Food allergies that cause a reaction when the patient comes in contact with even a tiny amount of a certain food. Allergic reactions occur either on the skin or in the stomach and intestines. Symptoms range from swelling and hives to vomiting and diarrhea.

Allergic rhinitis refers to an allergic reaction that causes sneezing and/or runny nose, itchy eyes, or itchiness or tingling on the roof of the mouth. This kind of allergy can be seasonal or year round. The seasonal kind is commonly known as hay fever and is usually caused by pollens. Ongoing symptoms are usually caused by exposure to indoor allergens, such as pets, dust mites, or indoor molds.

Atopic (no contact) and contact dermatitis caused by allergens causes skin conditions, such as rashes, hives (urticaria), or eczema. The allergens are sometimes easy to identify, like when someone has been hiking and three days later develops a case of poison ivy. Other times, it can be difficult to pin down the culprit. It could be medications, cosmetics, insect stings, foods, animals, or chemicals. Though not a cause, emotional stress over the appearance of symptoms can aggravate allergies.

Asthma is a chronic allergic disease that causes frequent episodes of wheezing, coughing, shortness of breath, and/or a tightness in the chest. Asthma can be mild, characterized by a chronic cough caused by airway muscle spasms. It can also cause life-threatening attacks that stop an individual's ability to breathe. Asthma can be non-allergic or allergic. Either way, it is common for people with asthma to also suffer from allergies. Both are set off by certain triggers, which could be anything. Common triggers include airborne substances like pollen or mold spores, respiratory infections like the common cold, physical activity, cold air, and air pollutants, such as smoke.

Anaphylaxis is the most serious kind of allergic reaction. It is potentially fatal because it often affects many parts of the body at the same time. Fortunately, it is rare. The allergens causing anaphylaxis are the same as any other allergy, but the reaction is extreme. It can cause a dangerous drop in blood pressure, loss of consciousness, swelling of the throat, and difficulty breathing. Treatment, which is an injection of epinephrine (adrenaline) with an EpiPen, must be immediate.

Allergy specialists can also choose to specialize. Some specialize in certain types of allergies or conditions, such as asthma or food allergies. There are also opportunities to work with patients with rare and/or potentially life-threatening issues, such as organ transplant rejection or allergic responses to water or sunlight.   Others specialize in certain populations, such as children. This is the largest and fastest growing group of allergy and asthma sufferers, with one out of five children having a food allergy and/or asthma. Another large group is adults with occupational lung disease, caused by inhaling specific irritants.

Diagnosis

Diagnosing an allergy is a multistep process that looks at the whole picture. It starts with a physical examination, which may include breathing tests and stress tests. The allergist will be looking for any anomalies in physical condition as well as allergic symptoms.

Next, the allergist gets personal. There will be an in-depth discussion of medical history, covering both overall health and symptoms that may be allergy related. The allergist will also ask about family history. There will be many questions about lifestyle, such as where the patient works and plays, to pinpoint any possible environmental sensitivities. There will be a list of possible allergens to check off, from fabrics and cosmetics to medications and foods.

Allergy specialists never assume they know what kind of allergen is causing symptoms. They are usually able to narrow down the possibilities before ordering specialized diagnostic tests. That is important, because testing for a full spectrum of allergens can result in many false positives.

There are two basic types of allergy tests: skin tests and blood tests.

The most common type of allergy test is the skin test. It is also known as a scratch test because a tiny bit of potential allergen is scratched or pricked onto the skin. This kind of test is quick and can be done in the allergist's office. Results can be seen within 15 minutes. If the area turns red and swells to look like a mosquito bite, the test is positive, meaning the patient has a sensitivity to that particular allergen. Results are also accurate, so treatment can be planned in the same visit.

Less common is the blood test. These are typically reserved for situations in which the patient is unable to tolerate a skin test. For example, the patient might have very sensitive skin or the patient might be on medication that would affect the skin's reaction. The advantage of a blood test is the ability to test for several allergens at once. The disadvantage is the expense – it can cost hundreds of dollars. A blood test is usually not done in the doctor's office because it must be processed in a laboratory. It usually takes several days to get the results.

Treatment

Once an allergist has a confirmed diagnosis, a personalized treatment plan is developed. The goal of the plan is to enable the patient to lead a normal, symptom-free life. A typical treatment plan will include measures to avoid allergens or triggers and recommendations for medications. The condition of the patient may be monitored and re-evaluated when necessary to ensure treatments are working.

Allergen avoidance is crucial for any patient. The first and most important step in treating an allergy or asthma is to identify the trigger. That is done with the tests. When the trigger is known, allergic reactions can be reduced or eliminated in most cases. If it is not possible to completely avoid the triggers, the allergist can suggest ways to decrease exposure and effectively manage the condition.

Medications can be common over-the-counter nasal sprays or eye drops. More serious allergies may need prescription medications in the form of pills or liquids that can calm immune system reactions and ease symptoms.

More serious or stubborn cases may require immuno-therapy, in the form of injections or sublingual tablets. Allergy shots containing the offending allergens are sometimes given to patients every week or two. By steadily increasing the amount of allergen, the immune system learns to accept it over time. It may take a series of injections over a period of several years to relieve all allergy problems. Sublingual medications are usually used to treat pollen and dust mite allergies. The first dose is taken in the allergist's office, then daily at home, by placing the tablet under the tongue until it dissolves.

The prescribed medication for patients prone to the most severe allergies is emergency epinephrine. Some patients need to carry an EpiPen with them at all times to control symptoms until they can get emergency treatment.

Asthma treatments usually require a prescription. The two most common are inhalers that fill the airways with anti-inflammatory steroids, and bronchodilators (also known as rescue inhalers) that open up the airways. If neither of these traditional treatments work, a medication such as Xolair may be used to reduce IgE levels, making patients less sensitive to their triggers. There are also drugs that help with long-term asthma control. They work by shutting down the effects of molecules called leukotrienes that trigger airway inflammation.

OTHER ALLERGY SPECIALISTS

MOST ALLERGISTS HAVE AT LEAST ONE allergy nurse and/or technician. By assuming some of the clinical tasks in a practice, the physician is freed up to perform more complex testing and handle more patients with serious conditions. The duties of these professionals will vary depending on the type and size of the practice, but in the private practice setting they may be asked to do the following:

- Take patient medical histories
- Administer pulmonary function tests
- Take vital signs
- Prepare examining rooms
- Conduct skin tests or collect blood samples for lab testing
- Prepare and/or administer allergy serums and injections
- Teach patients how to manage symptoms and how to use inhalers, nebulizers, and EpiPens
- Maintain patient medical records

There may also be some administrative responsibilities, such as scheduling appointments, ordering supplies, or completing paperwork needed for insurance billing. Conducting phone triage, especially during high-pollen seasons, may also be necessary.

TALES OF ALLERGY SPECIALISTS ON THE JOB

I Am a Specialist Allergy Nurse

"The best thing about my job is that no two days are the same. Allergies are more complex than most people realize. There are many different allergies and just about anything can be a trigger. A patient's experience can change at any time, too, making it even more challenging to manage the condition. But that is exactly what makes it interesting to me.

My patients are referred by the hospital. My job involves helping people manage their condition after they're discharged. Most have had scary events related to serious allergies. Imagine almost dying after getting stung by a bee for the first time. You are naturally going to be filled with fear and confusion. My job is to help them understand their condition and learn to cope with the fear as well as the condition.

My passion is helping patients enjoy a better quality of life, despite their condition. If I can do that for at least one patient, it is a great day."

I Do Research for a Teaching Hospital

"As an intern, I helped set up an audit of asthma deaths. I was stunned by the results and couldn't stop wondering what could have been done to save some of those lives. Today, I study genes and their relationship to the development of asthma and severe allergies. What I am looking for is the possibility of prevention through applied epigenetics. I also run clinical trials using innovative antibodies created in the lab. Many of our grants come from industry organizations seeking new medications.

This is a teaching hospital, so I also teach students and healthcare professionals who are interested in learning more about the specialized area of allergies and asthma. This gives me the unique opportunity to share what I've learned, which will hopefully lead to more successful outcomes in the field.

The research arena offers tremendous opportunities. I was attracted to this field because it clearly has so far to go. It is still in its infancy – what we don't yet know about allergies and asthma is far greater than what we have learned so far. It can be a great career field if you have a sharp, analytical mind and enjoy investigating medical causes and effects. Knowing that we can develop treatments capable of reversing these chronic diseases is exciting and rewarding."

I Am a Pediatric Allergist

"As a resident, I pursued pediatrics because I really enjoyed working with kids as a medical student. Kids are the bravest people I know. After seeing two children dying from asthma, I added a subspecialty in allergy medicine to my training. Since patients are primarily seen in an outpatient setting, I got together with two friends from med school and started a pediatric allergy clinic which we own as partners.

It's a great job, with so many interesting and varied opportunities to help kids. The most common conditions I treat include asthma, chronic cough, and food allergies. The demand for our services was huge right from the start and now, after less than five years, we are working at full capacity, and trying to hire another doctor and nurse. There are simply not enough trained allergists to keep up with the growing number of kids with allergies and asthma.

I love working with kids. I want them to have a normal life, playing with their friends and not feeling like they're defective. The best thing ever is receiving a thank you note from a parent whose child is happier and healthier."

PERSONAL QUALIFICATIONS

ALLERGISTS ARE THINKERS AND HELPERS. Through many years of training, they acquire the technical expertise needed to test, diagnose, treat, and manage the wide array of allergy disorders. There are also certain characteristics that effective allergists possess that help them think their way to successful outcomes.

Successful allergists like searching for facts that can lead to an accurate diagnosis. They possess the critical thinking skills needed to look beyond the standard tests for answers. They can analyze a patient's medical history and find clues that others might miss. Allergy-related problems can be far more complicated than most well-trained healthcare professionals can handle. Allergists rely on their analytical skills to identify and manage unusual allergic reactions.

Allergists also possess a high degree of intellectual curiosity. A plethora of allergy diseases have appeared in recent years and new ones seem to be showing up all the time. The best allergists do not rely on the basic knowledge they learned in school. They are avid readers, eager to learn about the new diseases being identified or the many clinical drug trials that may soon help them treat their patients more effectively.

Most people go into the medical field because they want to help people. Allergists are no exception. Helping allergy patients requires compassion and communications skills.

The best allergists consider their practice to be more than a job. Their work is about making life better for their patients. They understand that without proper treatment, allergy sufferers miss out on many things most people take for granted. Many people also face the ever-present fear of severe reactions. Compassion is the driving force that pushes allergists to do whatever it takes to help people.

Managing allergies requires excellent communications and interpersonal skills. In the search for answers, allergy specialists often have lengthy, involved conversations with patients. In addition to discussing their condition and symptoms, they often need to ask personal questions about lifestyle issues. Every detail needs to be noted in the patient's file. When a diagnosis is made, allergists need to speak in clear terms patients can understand so they know how to cope with their allergies.

ATTRACTIVE FEATURES

THIS CAREER COMES LOADED WITH BENEFITS. Like most healthcare professionals, allergy specialists pursue this field of medicine to help people. Allergies can take a heavy toll on a patient's quality of life. Using a mix of psychology and science, clinical allergy specialists can improve a patient's life tremendously. Making such a huge difference is very gratifying.

Those involved in research also make a difference, and on a bigger scale. They are able to advance medical knowledge in a field that is still filled with unanswered questions. Their work has the potential to discover more effective diagnostic strategies and better treatments of allergic conditions. Someday, there might even be a cure thanks to a dedicated allergy researcher!

Allergy specialists get to build strong relationships with patients through multi-year treatment plans. They often take care of entire families because allergic conditions are often hereditary. Taking care of families over the continuum of their lives can be very enjoyable.

Beyond helping people, there are a number of favorable practical considerations. First, is the income potential. Like most doctors, allergists are paid well. In fact, they are currently experiencing the second fastest salary growth of all doctors. The average salary is $250,000 a year and there is potential to earn much more. They also get to keep more of it than some other kinds of doctors. Malpractice insurance, which can be astronomical for specialists like obstetricians and surgeons, is relatively affordable. Plus, all allergy specialists enjoy generous benefits.

There is a serious shortage of allergy specialists, which means that those entering the field will find plenty of job opportunities. The number of people with allergies is growing faster than the number of trained professionals to care for them. Patients are everywhere. You can choose to practice anywhere in the country.

Lifestyle is another big plus. Unlike some other medical fields, allergy specialists rarely (if ever) need to be on call to attend to emergencies. A consistent nine-to-five schedule is possible. Those in private practice can set their own schedule. Some do choose to offer hours later in the day and sometimes on Saturday to accommodate patients' schedules.

UNATTRACTIVE ASPECTS

LIKE MOST DOCTORS, ASPIRING ALLERGISTS face a long, tough road. It usually takes 13 years of training after high school to become a board-certified allergist who is ready to start practicing. It can be very expensive, and many students end up with a mountain of debt. The classes are hard, and most students experience stress and sleep deprivation while trying to keep up with the studies.

Allergy nurses and technicians only need to spend one to four years getting the necessary training, but they also have to study hard to master some difficult subjects.

The three years following graduation from medical school are grueling. Medical residents typically spend up to 80 hours a week in a hospital with single shifts routinely lasting up to 30 hours. By comparison, residents work more than twice as many hours as their educated peers in other professions – even in demanding fields like corporate law. Fortunately, this is the worst part of choosing to become an allergist. Once you are board--certified, the hours you work will be cut in half.

Most clinical allergists would prefer to spend all their time helping patients. Unfortunately, time must be spent dealing with nonclinical duties, like filling out detailed computer forms. Insurance battles can add time to the day. Trying to get prior authorizations and making the case for more expensive testing can be aggravating, especially when you are talking to someone on the phone who clearly does not have the training or authority needed to make out-of-the-box decisions. Those in private practice need to spend extra time on the business side of practicing medicine.

Treating allergic conditions is often a matter of educating

and motivating patients to make necessary lifestyle changes. Motivating people to change their behavior can be a frustrating exercise in futility. For some, exposure to pets can cause shortness of breath, rashes, and even severe asthmatic attacks. For others, consuming certain foods can lead to hives, swelling of the lips or throat, vomiting, diarrhea, trouble breathing, malnutrition, or severe abdominal pain. Yet, some patients will refuse to give up their beloved pets, or check food labels to avoid ingredients like gluten, eggs, peanuts, food dyes, lactose, or casein (a milk protein). You cannot force someone to follow a treatment plan, and it can be very disappointing to see a patient continue to suffer rather than get with the program.

EDUCATION

IT TAKES AT LEAST 13 YEARS OF postsecondary training to become a board certified allergist. It starts with four years of college as an undergraduate, then another four years of medical school. At this point, graduates have their MD (Medical Doctor) or DO (Orthopedic Physician), and are considered doctors, but those aiming for a career in allergy medicine are not finished yet. They will need three years of residency training and another two years in a fellowship program in allergy. The final step is obtaining certification.

Undergraduate Studies

Your college years will be focused on preparing for medical school while earning a bachelor's degree. Many aspiring doctors pursue a pre-med program, but it is not specifically required by medical schools. Other majors are acceptable, with a caveat. Your curriculum must emphasize the sciences and include classes in biology, organic and inorganic chemistry, anatomy, and general medicine subjects.

Undergraduate students will need to take the Medical College Admissions Test (MCAT). This standardized, multiple-choice exam is usually taken in the junior or senior year. Along with MCAT exam scores, admissions officers will expect to see letters of recommendation, high grade point averages, and an essay. Experience in the medical field is a plus, whether it is volunteer work or a paid position.

Medical School

The first two years of medical school will involve intensive classroom instruction and book study. Classes will cover subjects like anatomy, biochemistry, medical ethics, microbiology, pharmacology, psychology, and physiology. The third and fourth years include clinical training through rotations that expose students to a variety of medical specialties. Rotations take place at hospitals and clinics affiliated with the school so that students can gain experience within real medical settings. Under the supervision of experienced doctors, students learn how to take medical histories, diagnose medical conditions, and check on patients' conditions during rounds.

Residency

After graduating from medical school, you will need to complete a three-year residency program. At this time, you will need to decide if you want to work with adults or children. If you choose adults, your residency would be internal medicine. If you choose children, your residency will be in pediatrics. Residency programs are arguably the hardest part of becoming an allergist. Programs take place in hospital settings where 12 to 16 hour days of hands-on training are the norm.

At the end of those three years, you will need to sit for an examination from the American Board of Internal Medicine (ABIM) or the American Board of Pediatrics (ABP). By passing the exam, you will become certified in either internal medicine or pediatrics.

Fellowship

Once you are an internist or pediatrician, you are eligible for fellowship training in an ACGME (Accreditation Council for Graduate Medical Education)   accredited allergy training program. This is typically a two-year program in a teaching hospital where fellows can become highly specialized in unique cases involving allergies.

Certification

At the end of the fellowship, allergists are eligible to earn their subspecialty certification from the American Board of Allergy and Immunology (ABA). To receive the certification, you will need to take and pass another exam. This does not need to be done immediately. You have five years to prepare and/or retake if necessary. However, if you do not pass the exam within that time, additional education will be required.

Allergy Nurse

Nurses working within this specialty area are registered nurses (RNs) with advanced knowledge in allergy treatment and management. The most common route to prepare for allergy nursing is to earn the Associate Degree in Nursing (ADN), which can be completed in two to three years of full time study. It is the minimum amount of school required to become an RN. The ADN program is offered by community colleges, vocational schools, and some four-year nursing schools.

Upon graduation, ADN holders are qualified to sit for the National Council Licensure Examination for Registered Nurses, or NCLEX-RN. Since licensing is required to practice nursing, passing the exam is crucial.

Although not required, allergy RNs can also obtain certification in Asthma Education by the National Asthma Educator Certification Board.

Allergy Technician

Most states do not have any educational or certification requirements for allergy technicians. While there are some entry-level jobs that only require a high school diploma and some on-the-job training, it is very difficult to compete for those jobs without more formal education. Most employers (allergists and other physicians) want to see at least a one-year certificate or two-year associate degree in medical technology or a related field. Either way, coursework should cover basic medical topics, such as anatomy, clinical training, insurance processing, pharmacology, pathology, physiology, medical ethics, and medical terminology. Depending on the school, specialized courses in allergy medicine may be available.

Allergy technicians can add to their qualifications by obtaining certification. This is not required, but this kind of credential can move you to the head of the line when applying for jobs. Allergy technicians can choose from four institutions that offer certifications sanctioned by the Commission on Accreditation of Allied Health (CAAHEP) or the Accrediting Bureau of Health Education Schools (ABHES). The four possible certifications are Certified Medical Assistant (CMA), Registered Medical Assistant (RMA), National Certified Medical Assistant (NCMA), and

Certified Clinical Medical Assistant (CMA). The CMA carries the most weight on a résumé because it is the only one that requires formal education in addition to a passing test score.

EARNINGS

THE AVERAGE ANNUAL SALARY FOR A board certified allergist in the US is just over $250,000. Most allergists earn between $225,000 and $300,000, the median is $230,000. The median is the halfway point between the lowest and the highest salaries. These numbers reflect the base salaries only. Non-salary cash compensation, such as signing bonuses and other incentives, can add a few thousand dollars. In certain situations, such as group practices and partnerships, profit sharing can represent a significant boost in earnings.

How much any individual allergist is paid depends on a number of factors. The most important are experience, geographic location, and type of employer.

Earnings are greatly impacted by the number of years in the profession. An entry-level allergist with less than a year in the field, will earn an average total compensation of around $175,000. Five years later, that individual's earnings will probably surpass $200,000. Veterans in the field who have practiced for at least 10 years will be at the top end of the pay scale.

Salaries can differ from state to state, and also from city to city. For example, an allergist in California earns an average $280,000 a year, which is well above the national average. The range is between $250,000 and $325,000. Some of the variance can be chalked up to experience and work setting, but this is a big state and it matters where you practice. The average income for allergists in San Francisco is nearly $300,000 while just 186 miles away in Fresno, it is about $235,000.

Many medical professionals can expect higher pay in wealthy states on the West and East Coasts. States in between and particularly in the South have lower costs of living and usually have lower incomes to match. That is not necessarily the case with this career. In the field of allergy medicine, pay is often linked to the incidence of allergies within the state. Some of the worst areas for seasonal allergies are in Mississippi, Tennessee, Kentucky, and Texas. That creates demand for allergists that translates into good income opportunities. The salaries in these states do not quite meet the national average, but they are over $200,000. Considering that the average price of a home in any of these states is a fraction of one in California, relocation is worth considering.

More allergists are employed than are self-employed, but salaried allergists earn less than their self-employed colleagues. The average salaried allergist earns $225,000 a year compared to $345,000 for the one who is self-employed. Experience has something to do with this difference in pay. New allergists are unlikely to strike out on their own and start a private practice. They typically start out in a hospital setting where they gain experience, pay down their student debt, and build a reputation for quality service. Hospitals are not known for paying high salaries, especially to inexperienced doctors. In fact, the range of hospital salaries is 20 to 45 percent lower than that of other employers.

Other Allergy Specialists

An allergy nurse in the US earns an average of $60,000 per year. Differences in pay are primarily related to experience. Entry-level positions start at $40,000. The most experienced allergy nurses can earn up to $90,000 per year.

Clinical allergy technicians earn salaries in the range of $30,000 to $45,000. There are instances of allergy technicians earning much more, but that is unusual. The national average stands at $40,000, which is reasonable considering the minimal education requirements.

Benefits

All allergy specialists enjoy an array of benefits including paid sick days, paid vacation and holidays, medical and disability coverage, and life insurance coverage. In addition, there is often reimbursement for educational expenses. Some employers also pay for malpractice/liability insurance, which can present a significant expense for any doctor.

OPPORTUNITIES

FUTURE PROSPECTS FOR ALLERGY SPECIALISTS appear to be excellent for the foreseeable future.   For allergy doctors, and their nurses and technicians, there will be plenty of job opportunities and a variety of settings to choose from. The number of jobs for allergists should increase almost 20 percent over the coming decade. That is more than the national average for all occupations.

As good as that sounds, experts believe that the growing shortage of allergists could lead to even faster job employment growth. Some predict that the demand for allergy healthcare could increase as much as 35 percent. Many patients within the growing allergic population could be served by primary care providers, but that still leaves a huge number of people needing the expertise of a board certified allergist.

For at least five decades, the incidence of allergic diseases has risen dramatically, not just in the US, but worldwide. In the 1970s, only 10 percent of the population was affected by allergic disorders. Now, a large swath of the population has some type of allergic issue that needs attention. Children have been hit the hardest. Prior to the 1990s, no one thought twice about sending peanut butter sandwiches to school. Now they are prohibited in most schools. Food sensitization rates have spiked, and nearly 50 percent of school children have some kind of allergy. As with adults, some allergic reactions are minor, but others are deadly serious.

Some food related allergies were practically unheard of as recently as 30 years ago. For example, there is now a wide range of serious gastrointestinal, neurological, and nutritional problems caused by allergy to gluten. Some people still laugh off the gluten-free "craze," but to those afflicted with celiac disease, it is not a laughing matter.

In addition to food allergies, millions of children and adults are being diagnosed with rhinitis (hay fever), skin disorders, drug allergies, and immune problems, and asthma. Allergic disease is now the sixth leading cause of chronic illness in the US, with associated healthcare costs in excess of $18 billion. Asthma alone, which has tripled since the late 1990s, now affects more than 22 million Americans.

Many allergy disorders, especially the newest ones, need the expertise of a dedicated allergy specialist. A primary care doctor simply is not up to the task, but there is a growing shortage of allergists available. Of the 700,000 practicing physicians in the US, less than 5,000 are board certified allergists – not nearly enough to care for half the population. Consider that there are only a few hundred doctors in allergy residency training programs at any given time. Many of them are pursuing research roles rather than direct patient care. The result is a decline in the number of allergists while the demand for them is increasing.

For those who do choose a career in allergy medicine, jobs are everywhere because people with allergies are everywhere. Wait times to see allergists typically exceed 60 days in most cities. Many rural areas have no allergists at all. The job outlook is especially good for those willing to work in remote areas and states with the highest levels of airborne allergens. Some of these areas are so desperate for allergy specialists, they are willing to pay generous signing bonuses and top-level salaries to get the help they need.

There are also excellent opportunities for allergy specialists who want to travel and work temporary assignments. These locum tenens, as they are known, help combat the increasing shortage of allergists by filling in gaps during vacations and other leaves of absence and providing care to patients who would otherwise go without. Contracts are usually less than three months, with the option to renew. Pay is typically higher than staff salaries, and openings are available coast-to-coast with as little as 24 hours placement.

There are also non-clinical opportunities available for allergy specialists interested in research. One of the reasons that many new allergists go into research rather than clinical care is the huge demand for researchers. Recruiters are out in full force looking for more. Pharmaceutical companies are scrambling to come up with new and better medications to address the allergy and asthma epidemic. Government research facilities are looking for answers as to why so many people are affected by allergy disorders. There are many new allergic diseases that were unheard of until the late 1990s, and more seem to be appearing all the time. Government, university, and private research concerns want to know where they are coming from and what to do about them.

It will take an army of researchers to figure it out.

GETTING STARTED

WHEN LAUNCHING THEIR CAREER, most new allergists and their support team look for salaried jobs in group medical practices, clinics, and hospitals. According to recent surveys, new careerists rarely face any difficulty in finding full-time positions with these employers. Not surprising since the number of job opportunities exceeds the number of qualified candidates.

Many employers depend on educational institutions to provide a flow of job candidates. Recruiters regularly scout medical schools, hoping to be the first in line to hire fresh   graduates. Their point of contact is the school's career placement center. By visiting the center often, you can know when they are coming and make arrangements to connect with them. The career center will also post new job opportunity listings as they come up. The career center can also help you with career planning, résumé writing, and interview practice.

Recruiters also make good use of online job sites. Bigger sites like ZipRecruiter have thousands of jobs for allergy specialists posted at any given time. There are also job sites dedicated to the medical profession, such as NurseFinder and MDSearch. LinkedIn, the de facto social networking site for professionals, has a wealth of job posts and networking opportunities. It is also where the vast majority of recruiters hang out on a daily basis. If there is a particular hospital or clinic that you would like to work at, you will probably find job openings posted on their websites. Sometimes you can take a virtual tour and submit an application online.

Networking is one of the best ways to find jobs in the medical field. Talk to everybody you know about how excited you are to be licensed and ready to work. Your network of contacts should include faculty, residency and fellowship supervisors, and colleagues from any previous workplaces.

Your very best contacts will be your teachers. These are professionals who are often practicing themselves or are actively involved in professional organizations where they have many contacts. Make a concerted effort to develop good relationships with them so they will think of you when they hear of jobs that open up.

Join regional and national professional organizations and attend events and local meetings to make more contacts. Major associations often have job boards, but even if they do not, they will have calendars that show scheduled events. Conferences, seminars, and workshops provide excellent opportunities to meet people in the field and make connections. Membership also looks good on your résumé.

ASSOCIATIONS

■ **American Board of Allergy and Immunology**
https://www.abai.org

■ **Association of American Medical Colleges**
http://www.aamc.org/students

■ **American Academy of Allergy, Asthma & Immunology**
http://www.aaaai.org

■ **Association of Asthma Educators**
www.asthmaeducators.org

■ **National Asthma Educator Certification Board**
http://www.naecb.org

■ **The American Society of Allergy Nurses**
https://www.allergynurses.org

PERIODICAL

■ **The Journal of Allergy and Clinical Immunology**
https://www.jacionline.org

WEBSITES

■ **NIAID Summer Internship Program**
https://www.niaid.nih.gov/about
/summer-internship-program

■ **Accreditation Council for Graduate Medical Education (ACGME)**
www.agcme.org